CHRISTMAS DELICACIES

Augusta Tokens

Contents

Chapter One

Introduction

If you have celiac disease or one of those diseases caused by sensitivity to gluten, you may be suffering with debilitating symptoms and pain. Although, you don't have to suffer like that if you follow a gluten-free diet. You can have tasty, healthy, baked-goods that contain no gluten.

The body contains a complex and interlocking network to prevent disease. There is a network of organs and glands that are dedicated to warding off disease. But sometimes the immune system is mysteriously programmed incorrectly and attacks the healthy cells instead of harmful ones. These maladies are termed "autoimmune diseases".

Although the sources of auto-immune disorders are not fully understood, many medical professionals agree that the causes of these disorders are viruses that alter the information that is stored in a cell; radiation; certain chemicals, including heavy metals and chemicals; and drugs. They may also involve a relationship between auto-immune disorders and sex hormones since more women suffer than do men.

According to doctors: Celiac disease is caused by an autoimmune response to gluten, one of the thirty proteins found in wheat, barley, and rye. Gluten is present in many types of breads, crackers, pastas, and cereals. The gluten proteins in wheat, barley, and rye have the same chemical structure and share some of the same amino acids. Gluten may also be present in many other foods and

Humans as a species have difficulty assimilating the protein gluten. To get the protein gluten, the tiny particles must be broken into smaller particles, or amino acids, that can be absorbed by the body. Normal protein digestion involves a complete breakdown of the protein into small particles. Individuals who are not gluten intolerant don't appear to be affected negatively in the way of those who suffer from gluten intolerance.

But for those who are intolerant and get into their bodies, the undigested gluten protein gets absorbed into them.

Some people use small intestine lining as a replacement protein. However, the body doesn't make the protein lining and doesn't react to it as a protein source. Instead, the immune system attacks the protein particles and makes inflammation in parts of the small intestine. This can cause serious damage to absorption of nutrients in the small intestine and prevent it from working properly.

Normally, the small intestine is lined with villi, which are little "plush" carpet-like projections on a microscopic scale. These villi absorb nutrients from the food you eat.

In the absence of villi, the inner surface of the small intestine becomes rough and dry, making it hard for the body to absorb nutrients. As a result, the body does not receive the nutrients necessary for proper growth and health.

It's now clear that the disease is more common than previously assumed.

New research reveals that a common genetic disorder — celiac disease — may be one of the most common genetic disorders, with an estimated 1 in 133 Americans afflicted. That's more than 3 million people.

The condition is diagnosed by testing for three antibodies— anti-gluten, anti-endomysial, and anti-tissue transglutaminase—since these are present when a person is exposed to gluten but disappear when the offending grains are no longer consumed.

There are millions of people in the U.S. who don't have celiac disease, and they have found that following a gluten-free diet reduces or eliminates their gastrointestinal problems. In fact, in 2006, scientists were able to prove that non-celiac gluten sensitivity exists in up to 30 percent of the American population.

For this group of larger people, removing gluten is a popular way to eliminate health conditions ranging from abdominal pain to osteoporosis, and sinus congestion. Gluten-sensitivity has also been linked to conditions such as psoriasis, anemia, and asthma

Gluten-free eating should not be considered a temporary measure.

The body doesn't become less sensitive to gluten after elimination, especially not in the long-term.

The condition is likely to come back when gluten is reintroduced.

There is a glut of gluten-free foods available to the general public. This abundance makes it easier than ever for people to follow a gluten-free diet. Because the recipes in this book were created with available ingredients the most convenient.

Chapter Two

All the recipes

Caramel Pecan Bars

These rich and gooey cookies are like a pecan pie that you can hold in your fingers. They are from the Southern tradition, and every generation loves them.

Yield: 2 to 3 dozen

Active time: 20 minutes

Start to finish: 1 hour

Half a pound of pecan halves

1/4 cup brown rice flour

1/4 cup confectioners' sugar powder

1/4 cup sweet rice flour

1/4 cup potato starch

1/4 cup almond meal

1/2 teaspoon xanthan gum

1/4 teaspoon salt

1/2 pound unsalted butter, sliced.

1/2 teaspoon pure vanilla extract

1/4 tsp (2 ml) almond extract

3/4 cup firmly packed light brown sugar

1/4 cup (1/4 cup of the mix)

1/4 cup heavy cream

1: Preheat the oven to 375°F. 2: Line a 9x9-inch baking pan with two pieces of heavy-duty aluminum foil with a long piece of heavy-duty aluminum foil going up the sides of the pan. 3: Grease the foil

Combine rice flour with confectioners sugar, potato starch, almond meal, cornstarch, and salt in a food processor fitted with the steel blade. Blend for 5 minutes or until the mixture is a homogenous color.

Mince the garlic and process them in butter.

Add the eggs and vanilla to the work bowl.

4. Transfer dough to prepped pan with a large offset spatula. Using a floured fingers and an offset spatula, press dough firmly into the bottom of a 12 inch tart pan with sides about 3/4

minutes.

While the dough is rising, prepare the topping by combining the remaining butter, brown sugar, sugar, and corn syrup in a saucepan over high heat. Once the mixture comes to a boil, whisk constantly for 2 minutes. The topping is now ready for use.

6. Spoon over the crust, smoothing the top with a spatula. Bake for about 20 to 22 minutes.

When I want something to be ready when I get home, it's always best to prepare it in the morning. Otherwise, it is always best to cool completely in the refrigerator. You can pull up the sides of the foil over the top and cut the squares into small squares.

Variations

Use dark brown sugar, light maple syrup, and walnuts instead. 4. Original: There are several things that you can do to help students do their

Add 1/2 cup dried currants to the topping.

Although gluten is not present in this salt-free pizza dough, its structure holds the crust in shape as it bakes. By pricking the dough's surface with a fork, it prevents shrinkage in the oven.

Lemon Squares

This is a lemon and butter dish, which I've been making since childhood. This gluten-free adaptation of course also works with the traditional dessert, that has remained at the top of my list since I first created it. It is also a great last minute dish since most of us have lemons and other ingredients in our

Total: 2 to 3 dozen

Active time: 15 minutes

Start to finish: You can do an hour per day

1/4 cup brown rice flour

1 tablespoon of confectioners' sugar

1/4 cup of sweet rice flour is a good choice for the sweet rice noodles

1/4 cup potato starch

1/4 cup almond meal

1/2 teaspoon xanthan gum

1/4 teaspoon salt

1/4 pound (1 stick) unsalted butter, sliced

3 large eggs, divided

1/2 teaspoon pure vanilla

1 cup granulated sugar

1 tablespoon cornstarch

1/3 cup freshly squeezed lemon juice

1 tbsp. grated lemon zest

Confectioners' sugar for dusting

1. Preheat the oven to 350°F. Line a 9-inch-wide baking dish with heavy-duty aluminum foil, allowing the front and back to be rolled around the sides of the dish. Grease the dish with oil.

I'm mixing in different ingredients to be able to make a cake that is gluten-free and still moist.

seconds. Add butter to the work bowl, and process, using intermittent pulsing, until the texture resembles coarse meal.

Combine 1 egg, vanilla in a small cup, and whisk well. Drizzle liquid into the mixing bowl, and pulse 10 times, or until stiff dough forms. If the dough isn't coming together, add a teaspoon of milk to the liquid mixture, and pulse it 10 times, or until the dough

To 4.: Press dough into the bottom of the prepared pan. Bake crust for 20 minutes, or until lightly

While the dough bakes, make the dough's topping. Combine remaining 2 eggs, sugar, cornstarch, lemon juice, and lemon zest in a mixing bowl. Mix on medium speed for 1 minute.

6. On top of the baking shell, pour a layer of icing, then sprinkle with confectioners' sugar. Cool completely, and then cut into pieces.

Note: The cookies can be refrigerated for up to a week, tightly covered.

Variations

Replace the lemon, zest and juice with lime, and use a drop or two of green food coloring.

Instead of simply dusting the bars, melt some jam in the oven, and then glaze the bars with it.

Confectioners' sugar is often referred to as "confectioners' sugar" because it contains a small amount of cornstarch, which acts as a binding agent. If whipped cream is whipped with

Layered

I was a regular at the diner frequented by Mr. Rogers, even though I wasn't a child. I watched Mr. Rogers' special episodes as children and knew that a man who loved kids like I did was always there. When Mr. Rogers wasn't on the television, I

Yield: 2 to 3 dozen

Active time: 15 minutes

Start your workout now: 1 hour

1 cup chopped pecans

1 cup of Graham Crackers crumbs

1/2 cup gluten-free rolled oats

(a mixture of) 1 /4 pound butter and 1 14-ounce can condensed milk.

1 cup white chocolate chips

1/2 cup butterscotch chips

1/2 cup of shredded coconut

1. In order to bake, pre-heat the oven to 300 degrees Fahrenheit. Grease the baking sheet. Place the nuts on the sheet, and toast for five to seven minutes.

2. Combine graham crackers, pecans, and oatmeal in a mixing bowl. Combine well. Pat mixture into the prepared pan.

1. Add the sweetened condensed milk on the crust, and spread it into an even layer. 2. Sprinkle white chocolate and butterscotch chips over the milk and then top it with coconut. 3.

4. Bake for at least 25 minutes. If it browns quickly, take it out and cool completely on a cooling rack before slicing into pieces.

Variation

Substitute 1 cup of dried fruits or raisins instead of

A century after he invented modern condensed milk, a milkman from Ohio named Gail Borden, Jr., was credited with improving the milk production process that produced an economical, high-quality dairy product. Since its approval in 1858, Eagle Brand milk has gained a reputation for purity, durability, and economy.

White Chocolate Cacao Almond Blondies

The delicate white chocolate and crunchy pecans blend very well, creating great taste.

Yield: 2 to 3 dozen

Active time: 15 minutes

In an hour you could...

1 cup chopped walnuts

2/3 cup brown rice flour

[3/3 cup]

"1/2 teaspoon of xanthan gum"

Pinch of salt

1/4 of a pound (1 stick) unsalted butter, softened.

3/11 cups firmly packed light brown sugar

2 large eggs at room temperature

1 teaspoon pure vanilla extract

1 cup white chocolate chips

1. Place the walnuts on an oven-safe baking sheet, and bake for five to seven minutes, or until lightly browned.

2. Use 3 parts flour, 0.5 parts starch, 0.01 parts xanthan gum, and 0.1 part salt in a mixing bowl and mix

A recipe for an irresistible buttercream will include sugar and butter combined for a few minutes after beating them at low speeds with an electric mixer to combine, then increased to high speeds until the buttercream is light and fluffy.

4. When the eggs, one at a time, are added and the vanilla, the speed of the mixer should be slowed down to medium. Next, add the rice flour and mix. Stir in the nuts and chocolate, and spread the cake batter to an even layer in the prepared pan.

Bake a sweet bread for 40 minutes, or until a toothpick inserted in the center comes out clean.

She placed the chocolate in the cold oven, then closed it.

Variation

Substitute bittersweet chocolate chips for the white chocolate, and pecans for the walnuts.

Unlike milk chocolate, white chocolate has no solid paste and cocoa butter only as its base, which consists of sugar and milk solids. It melts easily, and must be melted slowly so that it won't clump.

These marble fudge brownies

I adore the combination of chocolate and cream cheese, and these brownies do both. They are always a hit, and can also be frozen until they are completely thawed.

Yield: 2 to 3 dozen

Active time: 15 minutes

Start to finish: 1 hour.

Rice flour

4 ounces of semisweet chocolate

4 tablespoons (2 sticks) unsalted butter

3 large eggs, divided

1 cup granulated sugar divided

1/2 cup brown rice flour

1/4 teaspoon xanthan gum

Pinch of salt.

1 (8-ounce) package cream cheese

1/2 tsp. pure vanilla extract

Before you add rice cereal to the mixture in the pan, preheat your oven to 350 degrees.

2. Melt chocolate and butter together over low heat. It will be a smooth liquid. Remove the pan from the heat.

Add 2 eggs, 3/4 cup sugar, and beat on medium speed for 1 minute Or add the following ingredients and beat on medium speed for 1 minute: 4 large eggs, 3/4

4. In a small bowl, mix cream cheese, remaining sugar, and egg until smooth.

and fluffy layers of chocolate. Spread chocolate batter over the prepared pan. Top with cream cheese batter. Swirl together with a small spatula.

5. Bake for 35 minutes, or until the top is springy. While it's still warm, cut your cookies into pieces.

Note: Brownies in an airtight container, placed in a freezer for a month, can be enjoyed for many months.

Variation

Add 1 tablespoon instant espresso powder to the chocolate batter to get a mocha-brownie.

The Aztecs first discovered chocolate and our word is from the Aztec

Chocolate was originally known as "xocolatl," which means "bitter water." Montezuma was rumored to have consumed up to 50 cups of chocolate a day.

Fudgy Hazelnut Brownies

I can't take my eyes off of you. My eyes are a little bit sticky, but only on you. If I could, I'd follow you wherever you go, even if it would make you mad.

The yield is 2 to 3 dozen

Active time: 15 minutes

Start to finish the hour

Rice flour

4 ounces unsweetened chocolate

1/4 pound (1 stick) unsalted butter

1/2 cup skinned hazelnuts

1/2 teaspoon pure vanilla extract

2 large eggs, at room temperature

11/4 cups sugar

1/4 teaspoon xanthan gum

Pinch of salt

Rice + 1 cup

3 tablespoons cornstarch

3 tablespoons unsweetened cocoa powder

2/3 cup confectioners' sugar for dusting

Line a baking sheet with parchment paper.

The best way to make chocolate is by melting a mixture of chocolate and butter. Melting chocolate and butter into one pot is a process that should be done in a saucepan.

3. Peel and chop hazelnuts. Toast them for 5 to 7 minutes, until browned. Set aside.

Combine vanilla, eggs, sugar, xanthan gum and salt in a bowl; whisk well. Then mix the cooled chocolate mixture with the dry ingredients using a rubber spatula. Spread the mixture over the brownies, and then sprinkle with hazelnuts. Smooth the top of the brownies with a rubber spatula,

5. Bake for 45 minutes, or until the top is dry and a toothpick inserted in the center comes out barely clean. Cool completely in the pan on a cooling rack, then cut into pieces. Dust squares with confectioners' sugar.

Variations

Substituting chopped hazelnuts for the whole nuts, chopped nuts for the chopped, and whole nuts for the whole.

Add a cup of miniature chocolate chips and a handful of peanuts to the batter and mix everything together well.

The cocoa powder will only solidify to a lumpy consistency if the container is exposed to humidity. You may remove the lumps by sifting the powdered cocoa through a fine-meshed sieve.

Chocolates

Here's a tray of cookies baked to perfection with a creamy peppermint frosting. And to make it even prettier, we've scattered some crushed candies throughout them.

Yield: 2 to 3 dozen miniature cupcakes

Active time: 15 minutes

Start Finish: 1 hour

3 ounces bittersweet chocolate, chopped.

1/3 cup heavy cream, divided

Amaranth flour

1/2 cup almond meal

3 tablespoons unsweetened cocoa powder

1/2 teaspoon xanthum gum

1/2 teaspoon salt

12 tablespoons (11/2 sticks) unsalted butter, softened, divided

2 large eggs

[1/2 tsp.] pure vanilla extract

1/2 teaspoon to 1 teaspoon mint oil

2 to 4 drops red food coloring

3/4 cup crushed red and white peppermint candies

According to a report on the front page of the Times, on September 12, 2013 a fire broke out at a home at 2724 West New York Avenue, Baltimore, Maryland, damaging a stove. The house had two bedrooms, one

Chocolate requires 80% power. You stir the mixture continuously until the chocolate is melted and then set it aside.

2. Combine amaranth flour, almond meal, coconut flour, xanthan gum, and salt in a food processor until it forms a dough.

Mixing bowl. Whisk well.

To soften the eggs for beating later, place the eggs in a medium saucepan half filled with cold water. Bring the water to a boil, then immediately remove from heat. Cover, and let stand about 5 minutes, then drain. Next, combine 2 cups of the confectioners' sugar, and 8 tablespoons of butter in an electric mixer at low speed. Once the butter and sugar are well combined

4. Put batter into prepared baking dish. Bake for 15 minutes, or until firm and toothpick inserted into the center comes out clean. Cool completely on cooling rack.

For the frosting, combine the remaining butter and sugar, and beat at medium speed with an electric mixer until light and fluffy. Add the remaining cream, mint oil, and if using, food color, and beat well.

When frosting is too thick to spread, add in additional cream by 1-teaspoon increments if necessary.

6. Layer chocolate, peanut butter, etc. over brownies and sprinkle it with crushed candy.

Cut into pieces.

Variation

For chocolate almond brownies, omit the food coloring and substitute toasted almonds for the peppermint candies.

Peanut butter and chocolate layered brownies

Frosting on top, topped with peanut butter. Chocolate on top again.

Yield: 3 to 4 dozen

Active time: 25 minutes

It takes 2 hours to get started and finish

11/2 cups (21/2 sticks) unsalted butter, softened, divided 3 ounces unsweetened chocolate

14 ounces bittersweet chocolate, chopped, divided 11/2 cups granulated sugar.

11/2 teaspoons of pure vanilla extract

1/4 teaspoon salt

4 large eggs

2/3 cup brown rice flour,

1/3 cup potato starch

1/2 teaspoon xanthan gum

1 cup roasted salted peanuts finely chopped

1 cup peanut butter 3/4 cup confectioners sugar

1 tablespoon whole milk

1. Heat the oven to 325°F. A 9 x 13-inch baking pan, be ready to grease the foil.

Melt and mix 3/4 cup (11/2 sticks) butter, unsweetened chocolate, and half of the bittersweet chocolate in a heavy saucepan. Set the pan aside on the stove until it has cooled down for 5-7 minutes. You can also do this in a microwave oven.

Mixing the ingredients will help keep the consistency of the cake smooth and allow the cake to have a lighter texture.

After four hours of baking, a toothpick was inserted into the center of the bread.

3. You will combine some peanut butter with 4 tablespoons of melted butter, and use the combination to make a creamy, delicious treat!

Spread some mixture over brownies, and chill them for 1 hour.

Add the remainder of the chocolate and the remainder of the butter to saucepan... Then stir until smooth. Pour the dollops of chocolate and melted butter over a layer of peanut butter in the dish. Let the chocolate harden.

7. Chill brownies, lightly covered with plastic wrap, for about one hour, or until the chocolate is hard enough to scoop.

1. Take brownies out of pan by pulling up on sides. Cut into pieces. 2. Bring to room temperature. 3. Serve

Note: Keep brownies in the refrigerator. They will stay fresh for up to 3 days.

Peanuts are used in cuisines around the world, but peanut butter, which is an original American creation, was first promoted as a health food. In 1904, the World's Fair in St. Louis

Muffins make a holiday meal more pleasing to the eye, nose and taste buds. The sweet muffins are a holiday side dish.

Christmas breads from different regions: · In Italy, a special bread called panettone, is eaten on Christmas day. · In Germany, Stollen is a fruit-stuffed bread.

Yeasty Matters

If you don't make yeast-risen breads because you are intimidated by working with yeast, then, you should try making yeast-risen breads now. In this article, I will share with you how to work with yeast, and I will leave you with more tips for

To create breads that rise, there has to be an interaction between some sort of flour, moisture, and a leavening agent. When we mix protein in wheat flour and water, we call into play gluten. Gluten is what forms and solidifies after being heated in the oven. This ability of gluten to make shapes like a dome from a liquid creates a wonderful texture. The problem for gluten-free bread is that it gets stiff after forming a solid shape and baking it. To solve this issue, recipes in this chapter include wheat flour as one of their ingredients. But you can also use gluten-free flours in

Yeast, like baking soda and baking powder, is an organic leavening agent. Yeast can be alive or dead, but it is an organic leavening agent. These are the same ingredients, just in a

Cold temperatures temporarily inhibit the yeast's action. By storing it in a refrigerator, yeast stays fresher for a while.

To make sure your yeast is fully alive, you must start with a process called proofing.

After boiling water in a pot, pour it into a bowl with the stirring spoon. If in the midst of the boiling process, you place the hot water onto the spoon, the water will cool off rapidly. You shouldn't stir the water with the spoon until after the water has cooled to around 110–115 degrees.

The proofing is to make sure the yeast has worked. If there is no foam, the yeast is dead, so discard it. #4. Take a few minutes to read your passage aloud. #5. Paraphrase the Original paragraph in a creative way. #6. Paraphrase the Original paragraph in

Bread's basic ingredients were not a mystery in the 17th century. However, it was not until 1796... when Amelia Simmons used pearl ash in her cookbook -

To prevent the dough from rising too quickly, or rising too late, the bread has to be kept at the right temperature. There are some tricks to create a warm enough temperature

Put a bowl of dough on a low-heat electric pad.

Put the bowl in the dishwasher and tell it to dry the dishes;

• Put the bowl in your gas oven to benefit from the warmth from the pilot light;

• Put your bowl in a cold oven over a large, boiling-hot pan.

Marvelous Breakfasts and Quick Breads

Quick breads are biscuits or quick cookies. Muffins are muffins, but they can also be called quick bread.

Quick breads can be made with instant or self-rising ingredients that can be prepared with little or no waiting time. They can be eaten as an alternative to yeast-raised breads. They can also be used in place of potatoes or rice as the base for stews or braised dishes.

Convertible Forms

The difference between muffins and quick breads is the amount of time one takes to bake and at what temperature they are to be baked. This chart can help the kitchen enthusiast if he/she wants to convert muffins to quick breads.

Baked Good

Time

Temperature

Standard Muffins

18–22 minutes

400°F

Oversized Muffins

20–25 minutes

375°F

Quick Breads

45-60 minutes

350°F

Pannetone

It wouldn't be Christmas in many Italian households without pasta, baci, cantucci, panettone, panettone spumante, panettone dello zucchero (lots

Yield: Makes 3 loaves

Active time: 30 minutes

Start to finish: 41/2 hours

1 cup brown rice flour.

1 cup tapioca flour

33/4 cups cornstarch

2 tbsp xanthan gum

2 (1/4-ounce) packages active dry yeast

1 teaspoon salt

1 cup golden raisins

½ cup of sweet Marsala

2

1 cup honey

4 large eggs, at room temperature

1 cup unsalted butter, melted and cooled; 2 tablespoons pure vanilla extract

11/2 cups chopped candied fruit

1 large egg yolk

Make sure you have three empty coffee cans

1) Combine the following in a mixing bowl: brown rice flour, tapioca flour, cornstarch, xanthan gum, yeast, and salt. Whisk well. Stir together 2) Combine the dry ingredients just made and the wine

Heat (100 percent power) 40 seconds.

Combine all the ingredients except the flour and raisins, in a mixing bowl, beating all the ingredients together at medium speed for 1 minute. Cut in the flour, and then add the raisins and candied fruit, mixing the dough thoroughly.

3. Cover the bowl loosely with a sheet of plastic wrap, and place it in a warm spot for about an hour and a half. Don't worry if the dough rises twice its original size, so long as it's a

Grease a standard sized can three times, each time with one part of bread dough, then cover loosely with plastic wrap. Allow dough to rise before using the doughnut pan.

While the dough rises, preheat the oven to 350 degrees Fahrenheit, and brush it with an egg-yolk mixture and bake for around 50 minutes. Allow the loaves to cool for around five minutes, then turn them out onto a wire rack to cool completely.

Note: Do not use bread that has gone stale. If you must remove it from the freezer, do not reheat it. Cut the bread in half, wrap and freeze for up to 2 months.

Variations

Use a substitute for the Marsala—brandy or a fruit liqueur.

You may substitute pure almond extract for the vanilla extract, soak the raisins in amaretto or other almond-flavored liqueur

Marsala, like Sherry (and Port), is a fortified wine, generally between 16-18 percent alcohol. It's made with three different varietals of Italian grapes, and it became very popular in England (during the mid-eighteenth century), which helped boost domestic production in Italy.

Stollen

Christmas breads are common in European cuisine. The bread is typically made with bread dough, which is very heavy and often contains dried and candied fruit.

Yield: Makes 2 loaves

Active time: 30 minutes

A great way to kick off your day is to macerate 1 cup black raisins for 1/2 hour.

1 cup golden raisins

1/2 cup dried cherries

1/2 cup [dried cranberries]

1/2 cup rum

1 cup brown rice flour is called for.

1/2 cup tapioca flour

33/4 cups cornstarch

2 tablespoons Xanthan

2 packets of active dry yeast

1 teaspoon salt

1 teaspoon ground cinnamon

1 teaspoon freshly grated nutmeg

Grind it into a powder

2 cups of warm milk (110–115°F) In my opinion, this paraphrase will pass as the original even after the

1 cup honey

4 Large eggs at room temperature

1 cup of unsalted butter, melted and cooled.

1/4 cup orange zest

1/2 tsp. pure vanilla extract

1 cup almonds

1/2 cup chopped crystallized ginger

1 cup icing

Note: Do note that fruits macerate overnight.

2. Combine an 8-inch springform cake pan with a diameter of 7 inches with a baking sheet in a cold oven (200 degrees degree Celsius or 392 degrees Fahrenheit). Add some plastic wrap to the pan and the bowl of

When you preheat the oven it reaches 350 degrees. Almonds cook for 5–7 minutes. Then you should put the pan in the oven.

3 Combine white flour salt, yeast, cinnamon, nutmeg, cardamom, and brown rice flour in a mixing bowl. Whisk well.

4. Combine the milk, honey, eggs, and butter in the bowl of a standard mixing bowl. With a hand mixer, beat at medium speed for 1 minute.

Slow down the mixer speed and add the meringue, fruit mixture, and the almonds and crystallized ginger. Beat for about 2 minutes.

1. Cover the bowl with plastic wrap. I had been told this by a pastry chef and this is the traditional method. The dough was

doubled in bulk at around 2 hours and 45 minutes and was done.

6. Divide the dough in half, and shape it into two loaves. Cover the loaves lightly with a tea towel, and allow them to rise for 1 hour, or until very puffy.

While a loaf of bread rises, bring the oven to 350 degrees Fahrenheit. Cook the loaf for one-and-a-half hours, or until hardened and brown. Then transfer the loaf to a wire rack to cool down for ten minutes. Once the loaf is cooling, frost that with Royal Icing.

Bread can be baked a few days ahead. It's good stored in a cool, dark, dry place.

Variation

Substitute bourbon or brandy for the rum.

Popovers

Popovers are a crispy treat, usually slightly sweet, that make any meal worth eating.

When you bake the brownies make sure that the oven is clear of all other dishes.

Yield: 1 dozen

Active time: 10 minutes

Start to finish: 50 minutes

1/2 cup white rice flour

1/3 cup potato starch.

1 cup tapioca flour

1/2 teaspoon salt

1/4 teaspoon xanthan gum

1/4 cup (10.5 fl. oz.) whole milk, slightly warm

4 large eggs

3 tablespoons unsalted butter, melted and cooled

1. Preheat the stove top at 400°F. Grease a 12-cup popover pan or muffin pan.

2. Use rice, potato, tapioca, salt, and

3. Combine milk, eggs, and butter in a blender, food processor fitted with the steel blade, or a heavy-duty stand mixer. Blend until smooth. Add flour mixture, and blend until smooth.

4. Pour out batter into prepared cups.

Be sure to remove the popovers immediately from the oven and wait about 3 minutes before serving.

Note: The batter can be made up to 2 hours ahead of time, and left at room temperature.

Blend again to distribute the ingredients before filling the cups.

Variations

Add 2 teaspoons of grated lemon zest and 1 tablespoon of finely chopped fresh rosemary to the batter.

 Scones

Scones are a type of cake, often served with tea & coffee, which originated in Great Britain. They are theBritish counterpart of biscuits

Yield: 1 dozen eggs

Active time: 15 minutes

Start: 35 minutes

1 cup flour

2/3 cup potato starch

2/3 cup tapioca flour

1/8 cup granulated sugar

1 tablespoon

1/2 a teaspoon of xanthan gum

1/2 teaspoon salt

2 big eggs, lightly beaten A: There is no obvious problem. The sentences are almost identical

Use 1½-cup heavy cream

1/4 cup sour cream

1 large egg beaten

2 tablespoons of whole milk

1. Place a clean, dry baking mat or parchment paper on a baking sheet

2. Add rice flour, potato starch, tapioca flour, sugar, baking powder, xanthan gum, and salt to a measuring cup. Whisk well.

3. Combine all the ingredients in another mixing bowl, and mix thoroughly.

4. To make dough into 12 mounds, and that the average height of dough on a baking sheet will be about 11/2 inches.

Egg, salt and pepper for the biscuits.

5. Bake scones for 14–17 mins or until browned and serve immediately.

Note: Biscuits can be made in advance and are great for refrigeration for up to one day. Reheat in a 300°F oven, covered with foil, for 5–7 minutes.

Variations

Add 1/2 cup dried currants or dried cranberries to the dough.

Add 1 tablespoon grated orange zest and 1 teaspoon grated lemon zest to the dough.

Substitute sugar firmly packed dark brown sugar for the granulated sugar.

Scones are traditionally served in England at afternoon tea with some sort of fruit preserves and clotted cream. This high-fat, high-flavor thick cream is easy to replicate in your own kitchen. Combine 4 ounces mascarpone with 1

A bowl of heavy whipping cream with a few tablespoons sugar added to it is all it takes to whip

Old-Fashioned Southern Biscuits

Although bread is a staple of the French diet, biscuit is the form of bread typically eaten at breakfast, lunch, and dinner in the Southern states (such as North Carolina, South Carolina, and Georgia). These gluten-free biscuits are incredibly light and tender and they are delicious eaten with butter and jam.

A dozen

Active time: 15 minutes

Start to finish: 30 minutes

1 cup of white rice flour

3/4 cup **potato starch**

1/3 cup tapioca flour.

2 tablespoons baking powder.

2 teaspoons granulated sugar

1 tablespoon xanthan gum

1/2 teaspoon salt

2 large eggs, lightly beaten

11/2 cups buttermilk

1/2 cup (1 stick) unsalted butter, melted

1 large beaten egg yolk

2 tablespoons whole milk

[**1. Preheat the oven to 375 F. Line your baking sheet with parchment paper or a silicone baking mat.**]

2. Combine baking soda, baking powder, potato starch, tapioca flour, xanthan gum, and salt in a mixing bowl. Whisk well.

3. Whisk eggs, buttermilk, and butter in a mixing bowl until well mixed. Add flour mixture and mix until smooth.

To assemble the dough, divide it into 12 balls, each around 2 1/2 inches in diameter. Mix the egg yolk and milk in a small bowl

5. Bake biscuits for 12 to 15 minutes, or until browned. Serve immediately.

The biscuits can be prepared to serve several hours in advance. And after reheating, they can be served at room temperature in a toaster oven, covered with foil.

Variations

Put the canned green chiles and grated cheddar cheese.

Combine 1 cup of brown sugar, 1/2 teaspoon of ground cinnamon, and 1/2 cup of chopped pecans in a plastic bag. Press the mixture onto the tops of the biscuits before baking.

Add 2 tablespoons chopped fresh herbs to the dough.

Add 1/2 cup freshly grated Parmesan and a teaspoon of Italian seasoning.

Add 1 1/2 cups chopped scallions. White parts and green tops, 4 inches of each.

"Biscuit" is the American word for biscuit, but that meaning came from a different source: John Palmer. In his

Journal of Travels in North America

Canada (1822) and by the year 1828, the definition of the confection was "a composition of flour and butter, made and baked in private families." The recipes for biscuit were found in all nineteenth-century cookbooks, especially those with recipes from the South.

Brazil

Like the breads of Italy, the Portuguese sweet bread is an luscious and light addition to any meal.

Yield: 11/2 dozen

Active time: 15 minutes

Start to finish: 35 minutes

1/2 cup (1 stick) unsalted butter, sliced

1/2 cup whole milk

1/2 teaspoon salt

2 garlic cloves

2 cups of tapioca flour

2 large eggs

2/3 cup freshly grated Parmesan cheese

A touch of freshly ground black pepper

It is prefect

When your batter is ready, add the butter, milk, and salt, and pour all together in a bowl. Using a wooden spoon, beat it together until mixed well. Then stir it once more so that it feels even.

Transfer mixture to a blender and blend on high until smooth. Add the eggs one at a time, making sure the machine is working well as you add and blending well in between each addition. Then add the cheese and the pepper, and blend well again.

If you're using a wooden spoon to mix batter, it would be best to use a small offset spatula to help you evenly distribute the batter.

5. Bake rolls for 18–20 minutes, or serve them immediately.

Note: Rolls can be prepared up to 6 hours -in advance and kept at room temperature. They can be reheated in a microwave oven. Use microwave on high for 20-second intervals until hot.

Variations

Substitute Asiago for the Parmesan.

When you're using a bacon-scented dough, add 1/4 cup finely chopped cooked bacon or ham to the dough

Add 2 tablespoons of chopped fresh basil and 2 tablespoons of finely chopped sun-dried tomatoes to the dough.

The way garlic tastes is determined by the way it is minced. Pushing the garlic in a garlic press or mincing garlic produces an even more intense flavor.

Basic Focaccia

Focaccia (pronounced foe-KAH-cha) is one of the world's great snacks. It contains a fair amount of oil, so it's not necessary to add even more oil or butter to enjoy it, and it's flat so it's perfect for splitting in

Yield: 1 large loaf

Active time: 20 minutes

Start to finish: 31 hours (approximately)

3

21/4 cups warm water (110-115°F)

1 cup sugar

21/2 cups

11/2 cups of tapioca flour

2 cups of soy flour

1 cup of millet flour

To make this batter

1/2 cup olive oil

1 teaspoon salty

Mix the yeast, water, sugar and brown rice flour in a regular mixer first, before adding the salt, and then whisk the mixture until it becomes foamy.

Once you have the gluten free xanthan gum, combine remaining GF ingredients. Whisk well.

3. Put the paddle attachment in the mixer and add 1/3 cup of oil, flour mixture, and salt.

Beat a low speed until liquid (bread milk) is incorporated to form a soft dough.

Knead dough at a medium speed for 2 minutes, then roll out dough and put it into the work bowl.

Using the dough recipe and technique described above, mix the ingredients until a soft ball forms. Then, cover the bowl with plastic wrap and place it in a warm (80–90°F, 25–32°C) area to let the dough double in volume. Depending on the weather conditions and location, the entire mixing process and the rise time can take up to two hours.

After 5 minutes, I turned the heat up to 450 degrees Fahrenheit and the oven on. I then pressed the dough into a metal pan. I covered the pan with a sheet of oiled plastic wrap and left it in a warm place for 30 minutes before I baked it.

I have made bread in the oven as it is described by a pizza chef and as it is also suggested in the cookbook "The Bread Book" by Jim Lahey. The dough is made from one-and-a-half cups of unbleached bread flour, 2 teaspoons of sugar, 2 teaspoons of salt, one teaspoon of yeast and one-and-a-half cups of water. The dough is then divided into four parts and

Note: Make ahead of time and keep in the refrigerator, tightly covered in plastic wrap.

Variations

Sprinkle the dough with   cup freshly grated Parmesan cheese, then use it to create a focaccia. Top the focaccia with chopped olives.

"Herb focaccia"

Meaty focaccia: Sprinkle the top with 1/2 cup chopped pepperoni, salami, or prosciutto.

A muffin is a muffin is a muffin.

Muffins are wonderful both at breakfast and as an after dinner bread, and I like the combination of corn with the flavorful cheese. You can also toast

Yield: 12 muffins

Active time: 10 minutes

Start to finish: 30 minutes

1/2 cup of brown rice flour.

1/3 cup potato starch

3 tbsp tapioca flour

1/2 cup yellow gluten-free cornmeal

1/2 tablespoon gluten-free baking powder

1 Tablespoon granulated sugar

1/2 teaspoon salt

¼ teaspoon baking soda

1/2 teaspoon xanthan gum

1 cup buttermilk, shaken well

1 large egg

5 tablespoons of unsalted butter

1 cup grated Cheddar cheese, divided

Preheat oven to 400 degrees, and grease 12-cup muffin pan. Or use paper liners and spray top of pan with vegetable oil spray.

2. Mixing rice flour, potato starch, tapioca flour, cornmeal, baking powder, sugar, salt, baking soda, and xanthan gum together in a large mixing bowl, add buttermilk, egg, butter and 2/3 cup of cheese and stir gently to wet the flour. The dough should be lump

remaining cheese.

3. Bake muffins in a muffin pan for 18–20 minutes.

Variations

Make a cheddar cheese and jalapeño Jack muffin, and stir 1/4 teaspoon cayenne into the batter.

To the mixture, add 3/4 cup of crumbled cooked bacon and 1/2 cup of finely chopped scallions.

Add one tablespoon Italian seasoning and one clove of fresh peeled garlic. Combine with the other ingredients.

There are many ways to keep food from sticking to your dishes in the kitchen. One of the ways is to get a vegetable spray. Although, this spray can make your counters sticky. However, next time, make sure to let the spray drip onto the counter. The excess can be wiped clean with an aluminum foil.

Parmesan Herb Muffins

Vegetable-based muffins can be made using any bread recipe as the base, but are most commonly used as a dish in place of bread. Since they use no yeast, they are ready quickly and can be used as a side for a quick dinner like roast chicken or grilled fish

Yield: 12 muffins

Active time: 10 minutes

Start "by finishing: 30 minutes"

Three and a fourth cup white rice flour

1/2 cup potato starch

1 cup tapioca flour.

2 cups of gluten-free baking powder

2 teaspoons Italian seasoning

1/2 teaspoon baking soda

1/2 teaspoon xanthan gum

1/2 teaspoon salt

Freshly ground pepper to taste

Three-fourths cup whole milk

2 eggs

1/2 cup olive oil

3 tablespoons of chopped fresh parsley}

Use freshly-grated Parmesan cheese.

2 garlic cloves, minced

Preheat the oven for 350°F. Then, grease and line a muffin pan with cupcake paper liners. Spray pan with vegetable oil.

2) Combine rice flour, potato starch, tapioca flour, baking powder and Italian seasoning

Add 1 cup milk, 2 eggs, oil, 2/3 cup cheese, and garlic to a bowl. Gently whisk to get lumps. Fill each cup with batter, and sprinkle with remaining cheese.

3. Make muffins for about 18–20 minutes. They should taste good for about a week and a half, so I recommend doing them on a weekend. Place muffin pan on a cooling rack for about 10 minutes, then serve either hot or

Variations

Add / half a cup of sun-dried tomatoes packed in olive oil, drained and chopped. Add the <u>olive oil from the tomatoes [to complete the olive oil used in the</u>

Substitute: Oregano for Italian seasoning, and lemon zest.

One of the most important aspects of preserving herbs and spices is to keep them in a cool, dark location. Because warm air can trouble their effectiveness, and light degrades their flavor. It's best to store these foods in a place where there is no strong breeze, like a cupboard. This is a common question that

Beer Bread

When I first saw the recipe, I knew I had to try it. It was so easy and

Yield: 1 loaf

Active time: 10 minutes

Start to finish: 50 minutes.

3 cups all-purpose flour

1 teaspoon of baking powder

xanthan gum

1/2 teaspoon salt

1/2 teaspoon baking soda

1 large egg beaten

1 (12oz) can gluten-free beer

1. Preheat the oven to 350°F. Grease a 9 x 5 x 3-inch loaf pan and line it with a piece of parchment or a silicone

2. Mix flour, baking powder, xanthan gum, salt, and baking soda together in a large mixing bowl; then, add eggs, and beer. Stir until batter is just mixed; it should have a lumpy consistency. 3. Pour batter in the prepared pan and bake for 18 to

Turn a loaf of bread over the counter and bake it for 30–40 minutes, or until a toothpick inserted in the center comes out clean. Then set it aside for five minutes, and you can either serve it still warm, or let it cool completely before serving.

Variations

For a sweeter bread, add 1/2 cup granulated sugar to the batter.

Add... Sun-dried tomatoes or oil-cured black olives or 1/4 cups of each to the batter.

Add one half cup of chopped scallions to the batter.

Add 1/4 cup chopped fresh dill to the batter.

Malt is usually used as an ingredient in beer. Beer usually uses malted barley or wheat, not sorghum. The most famous brand of sorghum-based or hybrid beer is Redbridge beer, which is the most widely available beer containing

Irish Soda Bread

This hearty rustic bread is a favorite of mine. It's also one of the easiest to make, and it comes to the table looking pretty with a bright shiny crust.

Yield: 2 (10-inch) loaves

Active time: 10 minutes

Start to finish: 50 minutes

21/2 cups brown rice flour

¼ cup potato starch

1/2 teaspoon tapioca flour

2 teaspoons granulated sugar

11/2 teaspoons baking soda

You'll need one teaspoon of xanthan gum

1/2 teaspoon salt

1/4 cup buttermilk

2 tablespoons unsalted butter, melted

1. [prepare oven for 375 degrees Fahrenheit](/en/cooking/boiling/set-temperature/set-temperature

(2) combine rice flour, (other ingredients), in a large mixing bowl and mix well Add buttermilk, and stir until batter is just combined. Dough must be a bit sticky.

Divide dough into two parts, and pat each part into a 6-inch round, place on prepared sheet, and cut an X the half-inch deep. Brush the cuts with butter.

4. Bake bread for 35–40 minutes, or until the tops are golden. Remove the bread from oven. Cool on a cooling rack.

Note: To serve bread, the loaf must be unpeeled. It is good to keep in a plastic bag loosely sealed at room temperature for 1 day, and up to 2 days.

Variations

A cake recipe that includes all-fruit raisins or other dried fruit will add a pleasant flavor and texture to baked goods.

Add 1/2 cup chopped scallions, white parts and 3 inches green parts,

Add "2 tablespoons crushed caraway or fennel seeds."

Baking is done by heating, folding, and turning the dough. You can do it with the heels of your hands, or place the dough flat on a flat work surface and roll it out with a rolling pin or hand-held rolling pin.

Cornbread

If you have a seasoned cast-iron skillet around, you can also bake the cornbread right in it. This is a versatile recipe that's also great to serve at a meal with any entree.

Serving Size: 6–8 servings

Active time: 10 minutes

Start with 30 minutes

1 cup of fine yellow cornmeal, gluten-free

2/3 cup white rice flour

1/4 cup potato starch

A tablespoon of tapioca flour

2 tablespoons granulated sugar

11/2 teaspoons baking powder

one teaspoon of xanthan gum

½ teaspoon baking soda

1/4 teaspoon salt

2 large eggs

3/4 cups buttermilk, well shaken

1/2 cup creamed corn

Butter, melted

1. Preheat the oven to 425°F. Preheat the oven to 425°F.

2. Mix together all dry ingredients in a large mixing bowl. In another bowl, beat eggs and cream together. Add dry ingredients to buttermilk mixture, and mix well.

3. Warm a greased pan in an oven. Then, spread batter in the batter evenly and bake cornbread in the middle of the oven for 15 minutes or until the top is pale golden and the sides begin to pull away from the edges of the pan.

Remove the cornbread from the oven after five minutes. Turn it out onto a rack.

Note: Cornbread is best eaten within a few hours of baking.

Variations

Add 1 cup of dried cranberries and 11/2 tablespoons of fennel seeds to the cup of sugar.

Add 1 cup of raspberries to the batter. To thaw frozen berries, simply toss thawed berries into a bowl filled with hot water.

Add 1/2 cup crumbled cooked bacon, and instead of butter, heat bacon grease.

Add 1/2 cup finely chopped pimiento to the batter.

Toss the dried apricots and Chinese five-spice powder into the batter.

If you like pecans, then add pecans to the mixture. Substitute dark brown sugar for the granulated sugar.

If you don't use buttermilk very often, it's a waste of money to buy a quart to use less than half in a recipe. Instead, buy buttermilk powder. It's shelved with the baking ingredients.

Almond Piecrust

This is my favorite crust recipe for fruit pies. It is sweetened with marzipan, and the aroma and flavor of the almonds meld with the texture of all sorts of fruit.

Yield: Enough for 1 (8 or 9-inch) two-crust pie, plus a little extra for the top-crust

Be motivated to get up and workout daily

11/2 cups of brown rice flour

1/2 cups potato starch

1/2 cup tapioca

1/2 cup almonds

1/2 teaspoon xanthan gum

1/2 teaspoon salt

There are 1 or 7oz depending on the brand

1/4 cup (1 stick) unsalted butter, room temperature.

1 large egg

2 tablespoons ice water

1/2 teaspoon pure almond extract.

Make a flour paste by combining: one and half cups of brown rice flour, one half cup of potato starch, one half cup of tapioca flour, one quarter cup of almond meal, one half teaspoon of xanthan gum, and one teaspoon of salt in a large mixing bowl

The size of the butter should be about the size of lima beans, and the dry ingredients should be coarsely chopped. If you use a pastry blender or two knives, you can chop the butter into dry ingredients until they are small pea-sized chunks

This can be done in a food processor with the steel blade fitted.

3. Combine egg, water, and almond extract in a small bowl and whisk very well.

Sprinkle the mixture over dough, use 1/4 tablespoon all at a time. Toss with a light fork until the dough is well mixed.

Put the dough in a bowl and mix it gently. When the dough has no more gluten, continue to mix it with a rolling pin.

If a 1 or 2- crust pie is to be baked, the dough should be formed into a 1 or 2 (5 to 6-in) round, rectangular, or free-form round. 4.

"pancakes."

Use both types of pastry dough when you make individual pastries like empanadas (fried fruit pies, popular in Spain) or pies, or when you make circle pies.

If you want to make a pie shell before it is filled with filling, prick over the bottom and sides with a fork or press in a sheet of aluminum foil and add dried beans, rice, or metal pie stones to the pie pan.

Bake at 375 degrees for 10 to 15 minutes.

As soon as the pies go in the oven, turn the heat down to 375, and bake for 7 minutes. Then turn the heat down to 350 and bake for 45 minutes more, or until golden brown. Bake the second pie the same way and invert it over the top, crimping the edges and cutting in steam vents.

Note: The cookie can be baked up to 3 days in advance and tightly cover with plastic wrap when frozen. The cookie dough sheet can also be frozen for up to 3 days in advance.

months.

Gluten-Free Graham Crackers

You need graham crackers to form the basis for graham cracker crusts. The graham crackers are a favorite topping for baked cheesecakes.

Although some of the crackers in this book have slightly different proportions of cheese to butter and additional sugar, these are the basic crackers you can use to make S'mores. They can also be used for other desserts like cream cheese crackers. [<

Yield: 16-20, depending on the size

Active time: 20 minutes

Start - Finish

11/2 cups brown rice flour

1/2 cup cornstarch

1/3 cup firmly packed dark brown sugar

1 tablespoon baking powder

In a medium sized bowl, mix 3/4 tablespoon of xanthan gum into a slurry

Teaspoon ground cinnamon

1/2 teaspoon salt

3/4 stick butter, 5 tablespoons whole milk

1/4 cup honey

One half teaspoon pure vanilla extract pure

Add to food processor bowl: 1 cup rice flour 1 cup corn starch 1 cup sugar 2 tbsp. baking powder 1/2 tsp. xantham gum 1 tsp. cinnamon

Combine milk, honey, vanilla, and eggs, then whisk well. Drizzle in the liquid and pulse a total of 10 times. When the dough is no longer crumbly, it's ready to use.

forms a ball.

3. Divide the dough in half, cover each half with plastic wrap, and flatten the dough into a pancake. Refrigerate the dough mixture for up to 2 days or until firm. It can also be frozen according to your taste

4. Preheat the oven to 350°F. Line the two baking sheets with parchment or silicone baking mats.

5. Roll out the dough using an oiled rolling pin and lightly dust with sweet rice flour. Roll both halves of dough into sheets that are 1/4-inch thick, Transfer the dough to two prepared baking sheets and cut each half into 10–12 pieces with a pizza wheel. Prick all over with fork.

When making brownies, bake a total of 15 to 17 minutes, or until the brownies become brown. Allow the brownies to cool completely on the cookie sheet placed on a wire cooling rack. Break apart the brownies at the scored lines, when no longer

Warning: Keep cookies in an airtight container, layered between sheets of waxed paper or parchment, at room temperature until ready to serve. Or refrigerate for about a half a month.

Variations

Substitute ground ginger for ground cinnamon.

"Sprinkle cookies with a mixture of 1/3 cup granulated sugar and 1/2 cup brown sugar."

teaspoon ground cinnamon before baking.

When measuring sticky ingredients like honey or molasses, spray the measuring cup with vegetable oil spray. The sticky ingredient will slide right out of the cup.

Raspberry Crème Fraiche Tart

Contemporary airline food includes interesting appetizers, hot meals, and even sweet desserts. There are even some new innovations that have emerged on the commercial airline food scene, including sweetened raspberries.

Yield: 6 to 8 bowls

Active time: 15 minutes

Start to finish: 3 hours, including time to chill 3 large eggs

1/2 cup granulated sugar

1 teaspoon pure vanilla extract

11/4 cups crème fraîche.

1 pint fresh raspberries, rinsed

1 (9-inch) pre-baked pie shell made from Basic Gluten-Free Piecrust

1. Preheat the oven to 350°F.

2. Whip eggs and sugar until thick and lemon-colored. Add a teaspoon of vanilla extract and two tablespoons of crème fraiche. Stir well, and place mixture in a double boiler. Heat it, stirring constantly, until hot and starting to thicken.

Place your raspberries into the pie shell along with the custard. Bake the pie for 10 minutes and then chill well before serving.

The pie can be frozen up to 1 day in advance, tightly covered.

Variations

Replace the raspberries with fresh blueberries or blackberries

Add 2 teaspoons grated orange and vanilla oil. If orange oil is available, use it as a substitute for vanilla.

When you're selecting boxes of fresh raspberries in the market, turn over the box and look at the paper on the bottom. The box should not have any red splotches on it, and

Chocolate Caramel Pecan Pie #paraphrase A: I agree with

"I think that every dessert should contain some chocolate, and this pie is like eating a candy bar. It combines crispy pecans and mellow caramel."

Yield: 6 to 8 servings

Active time: 20 minutes

Start to finish: Take 13/4 hours, including time to cool 11/2 cups granulated sugar

1/2 cup heavy cream

In a large bowl, blend together the butter, bourbon and salt.

2 large eggs

1 cup pecans, toasted at 350°F for 5 minutes 4 ounces bittersweet chocolate, melted</

1

1. Combine equal parts sugar and water in a small saucepan over medium heat. Cook, stirring occasionally with a long spoon, until the mixture boils. Turn off heat and carefully pour 1/3 cup cream. Stir with a long spoon. Pour caramel back into saucepan and cook over low heat for 2 minutes.

Pour the mixture of peanut butter, honey, and coconut oil. Allow it to cool for 10 minutes.

2. Preheat the oven to 400°F.

3. Beat butter, bourbon whiskey, and eggs into a caramel until smooth. Stir in pecans.

Spoon chocolate pudding into pie shell and pour pecan pie filling on top. Bake for 15 minutes, then reduce heat to 350°F and bake 15 more minutes.

Allow the pie to cool on a wire rack until it's lukewarm.

The pie can be made a day ahead and can be refrigerated, tightly covered. Bring it to room temperature before serving.

Variations

Substitute rum or brandy for the bourbon.

Substitute walnuts, almonds or pine nuts for the pecans.

It is not difficult to make caramel, but one pitfall is allowing the sugar to actually reach the darkest brown before removing the pan from the heat. Be very careful while cooking the syrup, removing the pan from the heat when the sugar caramelizes to a medium dark brown colour; it will continue to cook.

Peanut Butter Cheesecake

The holidays are a special time when families often come together, and this dessert that features a ganache made with chocolate and peanut butter is a favorite among children.

Yield: It yields 8 to 10 servings.

Active time: 20 minutes

Start to finish: 2 hours, including time to chill 11/2 cups crumbs

6 tablespoons unsalted butter

1 cup sugar

1 cup creamy commercial peanut butter

The most important thing to know about creams is that they must ALWAYS be softened to work right.

Use 1 teaspoon of pure vanilla extract.

One-third cup heavy cream

8 ounces bitter chocolate, chopped

1. Make a batch of crumbs for the pie crust, and mix them with butter, a pinch of salt, and a tablespoon of sugar. Press this mixture into the bottom and up the sides of a 9-inch pie plate. Bake for 8 to 10 minutes, or until lightly browned.

We beat peanut butter and sugar with two electric mixers on medium speed until fluffy. We then added cream cheese, the remaining butter, and vanilla, and beat until combined. We whipped 3/4 cup cream on medium speed until medium-soft peaks form. We then folded the whipped cream into the peanut butter mixture until it was thoroughly combined. We kept the peanut butter cream

3. While the chocolate is still liquid, stir in the cream and the remaining chocolate.

4. Remove mousse from fridge. Beat on low speed, with an electric mixer, for a few minutes.

at least 5 minutes, or until light and fluffy. Cover chocolate layer with peanut butter mousse and distribute it evenly with a spatula. Place remaining chocolate in a pastry bag fitted with the small tip or in a plastic bag with small hole at one corner. Drizzle it decoratively over mousse. Chill until ready to serve.

The pie can be prepared in advance and refrigerated.

Variation

Substitute peanut butter for the commercial almond butter.

Pumpkin Pecan Cheesecake Bites

Miniature cheesecake bites are a great addition to any dessert buffet.

These moist and rich treats are flavored like a traditional pumpkin pie, with a base made of crispy pecans.

Yield: Makes over 2 dozen

Active time: 20 minutes

Start to finish: 6 hours, including time to chill 11/2 cups toasted pecans

3 tablespoons honey

3 tablespoons butter, melted

11/4 teaspoon ground cinnamon

Your workout program must be designed.

11/4 cups granulated sugar

4 large eggs

1 can pure pumpkin

1/2 cup half-and-half

2 tablespoons of brown rice flour

1 teaspoon vanilla extract

3/4 teaspoons ground ginger

1/4 teaspoon salt

Sweetened whipped cream

1. Preheat the oven to 350°F. Lightly grease a 9x13 inch baking pan.

Combine pecans, brown sugar, and 1/4 teaspoon cinnamon. Press into a greased 7-cup round tube pan so that it comes in one solid piece.

mix into the bottom of the pan, and bake for 15 minutes. Cool completely.

3. Mix cream cheese and sugar together in a mixing bowl, and then beat until smooth. In a separate bowl, mix pumpkin, half-and-half, rice flour, vanilla, ginger, salt, and the remaining cinnamon. Pour the pumpkin mixture on top of the cream

In order to create a large cheesecake, set aside the smaller baking pan and pour enough boiling water into the larger pan until it reaches at least 1 half deep. Afterward, the cheesecake can then be placed inside the water bath to cool. It is a better way to make smaller cheesecakes - if you keep the water bath filled.

Using a small scoop, remove the cake from the cake tin by pulling up on the sides of the tin. Cut the cake into circles using a biscuit cutter. Fill each circle with whipped cream.

The cheesecake can be made 1 day or 2 days in advance. Do not add the whipped cream until just prior to serving.

Variation

Substitute hazelnuts, walnuts, or almonds for the pecans.

Be careful when shopping for pumpkin. Right next to the boxes of canned pumpkin, which is great because it's always pure pumpkin, and there's no gluten in it, are cans of pumpkin pie fill which has sugar, spices, evaporated milk and usually wheat flour added.